Vibrant Mediterranean Diet Guide

Simple & Appetizing Dishes for Your Diet

Joseph Bellisario

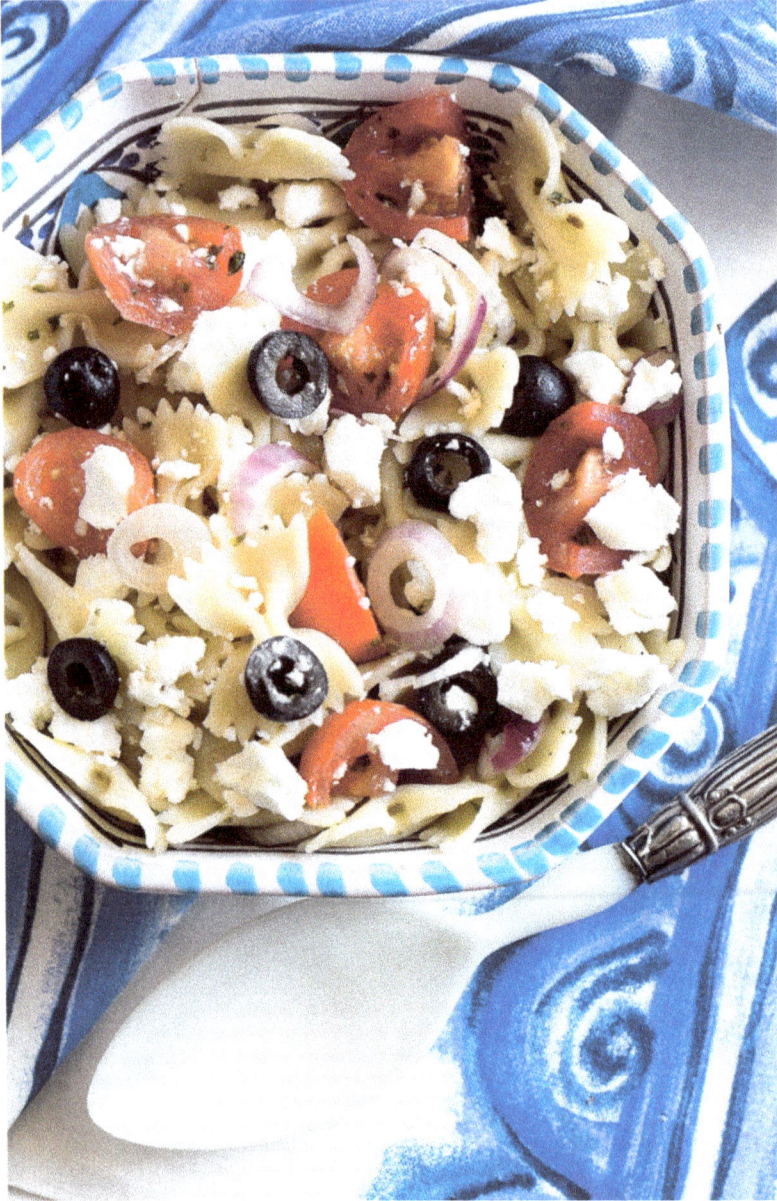

indirect, which are incurred as a result of the use of information contained within this document, including, but not limited to, — errors, omissions, or inaccuracies.

TABLE OF CONTENTS

Chicken, leek, and pea pasta bake

Ingredients

- 200g of cooked chicken
- 1 tablespoon butter
- 225ml of milk
- 150g of frozen peas
- 350g of pasta
- 250g of ricotta cheese
- Olive oil
- 2 leeks
- 2 cloves of garlic
- 60g of Parmesan cheese
- 100ml of chicken stock
- 100ml of white wine

Directions

1. Preheat the oven to 350°F and grease your baking dish.
2. Then, cook the pasta in a large pan of boiling salted water, let be undercooked.
3. Drain any excess water.
4. Return to the saucepan and coat with a drizzle of olive oil.

5. Place butter in a frying pan, fry the leeks for 10 minutes.

6. Add the garlic, stock, and wine and cook for 10 minutes.

7. Add the peas, cook for 30 seconds, stirring once.

8. Add the leek mixture, chicken, milk, and 2/3 of the ricotta to the drained pasta.

9. Let combine.

10. Season with salt and pepper.

11. Spoon the pasta mixture into the baking dish.

12. Top with the remaining ricotta, grate over the Parmesan, and drizzle with olive oil.

13. Bake for 25 minutes.

14. Serve and enjoy.

Sweet leek, ricotta, and tomato lasagna

Ingredients

- 1 packet of lasagna sheets
- 4 leeks, thinly sliced
- 75g of fresh parmesan, grated
- 2 red onions, thinly sliced
- Sea salt
- 250g of spinach
- Olive oil
- 350g of ricotta
- Freshly ground black pepper
- 1-liter tomato sauce
- 125g of mozzarella ball

Directions

1. Preheat your oven ready to 350°F.
2. Heat a large saucepan, add a splash of olive oil when hot.
3. Add the leeks together with the sliced red onions, and sweat, for 10 minutes.
4. Add the chopped spinach and briefly cook until wilted down.

5. Drain off any excess.

6. Mix the ricotta into the leek and onion mixture.

7. Season with a tiny pinch of salt and pepper.

8. Spoon a quarter of the tomato sauce into the bottom of 6 individual ovenproof dishes.

9. Cover with sheets of lasagna.

10. Then, spread half the leek and ricotta mixture over the lasagna.

11. Add the remaining tomato sauce. Repeat with all the lasagna sheets, leek and ricotta mixture, and the remaining tomato sauce.

12. But finish with a layer of lasagna sheets.

13. Tear the mozzarella into small pieces and dot over the top of the lasagna.

14. Sprinkle with the Parmesan.

15. Bake the individual lasagna for 30 minutes.

16. Serve and enjoy.

Sausages with pan cooked chutney and leek mash

Ingredients

- 5cm piece of fresh ginger, grated
- 1kg of potatoes, peeled and halved
- 3 tablespoons of balsamic vinegar
- Olive oil
- 2.5cm piece cinnamon stick
- 2 leeks, sliced
- 1 handful of fresh cranberries
- 2 red onions, cut into thin wedges
- 8 pork sausages
- 200ml of milk
- Extra virgin olive oil
- 1 sprig fresh sage, leaves picked

Directions

1. Begin by cooking the potatoes in simmering water for 15 minutes.
2. Drain, cover and set aside.
3. Add olive of oil to a separate saucepan with the leeks.
4. Sweat gently for about 5 minutes.

5. Then, add bring to the boil the milk.

6. Turn off the heat, then add to the potatoes.

7. Mash and season to taste. Cover and set aside.

8. Preheat the grill to medium.

9. Add a splash of olive oil to a frying pan over a medium heat.

10. Fry the sage leaves until crisp, set aside.

11. Sauté the onions for 5 minutes, add the cranberries together with the cinnamon and a splash of water.

12. Let simmer for 15 minutes, stirring, until the onions are soft.

13. Add the ginger together with the vinegar, cook for 30 seconds. Season.

14. Place the sausages under the grill for 15 minutes, turning frequently, until cooked.

15. Serve and enjoy with the chutney, mash, and sage leaves.

Slow roasted balsamic tomatoes with baby leeks and basil

Ingredients

- 12 plum tomatoes
- 200ml of balsamic vinegar
- 4 cloves garlic
- 2 tablespoons of extra virgin olive oil
- Freshly ground black pepper
- 1 handful of fresh basil
- 12 fresh bay leaves
- 12 baby leeks
- Sea salt

Directions

1. Preheat the oven to 325°F.
2. Score the tops of the tomatoes with a cross.
3. Take an earthenware dish that the tomatoes will fit snugly into.
4. Sprinkle the garlic and basil all over the bottom.
5. Stand the tomatoes next to each other in the tray, on top of the garlic and basil, then push the bay leaves well into the scores in the tomatoes, season.

6. Lay the leeks on a board.

7. Sprinkle generously with salt and pepper.

8. Squeeze the seasoning into the mixture by pressing with a rolling pin.

9. Weave the leeks in and around the tomatoes.

10. Pour over the balsamic vinegar, drizzle over the olive oil.

11. Let bake in the preheated oven for 1 hour.

12. Remove the bay leaves.

13. Serve and enjoy over pasta.

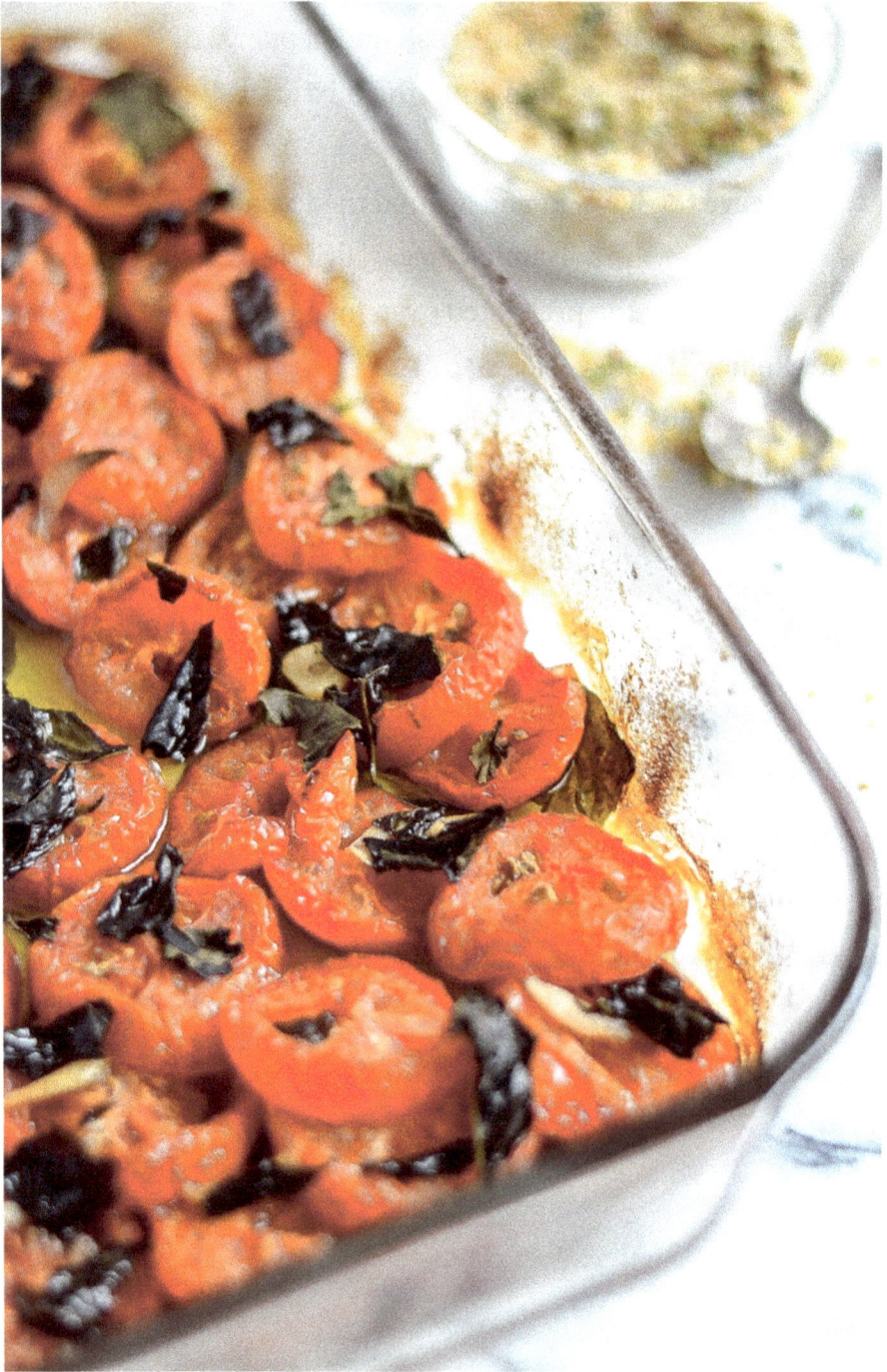

Roasted concertina squid with grilled leeks and a warm chorizo dressing

Ingredients

- 4 medium-sized squid
- Extra virgin olive oil
- 100g of chorizo sausage
- 2 cloves garlic
- 8 baby leeks
- 3 tablespoons of balsamic vinegar
- Olive oil
- Juice from one lime
- 1 sprig fresh rosemary
- 2 lemons, halved
- Sea salt
- Freshly ground black pepper
- 1 bulb fennel
- 1 radicchio, leaves separated

Directions

1. Firstly, preheat a griddle pan.

2. Then, preheat your oven ready to 475°F.

3. Parboil the baby leeks for 3 minutes in a pan of boiling salted water.

4. Drain in a colander, then let steam dry.

5. Dress with some olive oil and a pinch of sea salt.

6. Griddle, and cook the leek until marked with the griddle lining, add the fennel wedges, chargrill these dry on both sides until they are also marked.

7. Add the radicchio leaves and dry grill to wilt.

8. Put the leeks fennel and radicchio into a large bowl.

9. Heat a frying pan with olive oil.

10. Fry the chorizo until the fat renders out, then add the rosemary with the garlic, toss briefly and remove.

11. Add the balsamic vinegar with some lemon juice to the pan, mix.

12. Drizzle some olive oil over each squid, sprinkle with some salt and pepper, toss.

13. Preheat an ovenproof pan with bit of olive oil, toss the reserved tentacles in the oil for 1 minute.

14. Add all the squid and whack the pan in the preheated oven briefly until cooked.

15. Pour the chorizo dressing over your chargrilled veggies with a squeeze of lemon juice.

16. Serve and enjoy.

Roasted baby leek with thyme

Ingredients

- 2 cloves garlic
- 20 baby leeks
- 1 teaspoon of chopped fresh thyme leaves
- Olive oil
- Red wine vinegar

Directions

1. Preheat your oven ready to 400°F.
2. Place the leeks in a pan of boiling salted water for 3 minutes.
3. Drain any excess water.
4. Toss with olive oil, chopped thyme leaves, a splash of red wine vinegar, and the garlic in a bowl.
5. Arrange the leeks in one layer in a baking tray.
6. Let roast in the preheated oven for 10 minutes or so until golden.
7. Serve and enjoy.

Roasted chicken breast with pancetta, leeks, and thyme

Ingredients

- Olive oil
- 1 chicken breast
- 1 pinch of sea salt
- 2 whole sprigs thyme
- 1 pinch of freshly ground black pepper
- 1 large leek
- 1 small swig of white wine
- 4 slices of pancetta

Directions

1. Preheat the oven to 400°F.
2. Place 1 chicken breast in a bowl.
3. Add the leek, leek leaves, fresh thyme, pinch of salt, black pepper, swig of white wine, and olive oil, toss.
4. Place the leek with the flavorings into the tray.
5. Wrap the chicken breast in 4 slices of pancetta.
6. Drizzle with olive oil, place whole thyme sprigs on top.
7. Let cook for 35 minutes in the preheated.

Chargrilled marinated vegetables

Ingredients

- 2 red peppers
- 1 clove garlic
- 1 large bunch of fresh basil
- 2 tablespoons of herb
- 2 yellow peppers
- 2 medium courgettes
- 1 bulb fennel
- 1 aubergine
- 8 baby leeks
- Freshly ground black pepper
- Sea salt
- Extra virgin olive oil

Directions

1. Griddle pan, place all peppers on until black on all sides.
2. Grill the courgette with the fennel together for 1 minute on each side.
3. Transfer to a clean tea towel in one layer.
4. Chargrill the aubergine slices, turn 4 times until marked.

5. Transfer to the tea towel.
6. Boil the baby leeks in salted water until cooked.
7. Drain, then rub with bit of olive oil, and chargrill until lightly marked.
8. Place all the vegetables into a large bowl.
9. Bash some basil leaves in a pestle and mortar with a pinch of seasoning until a smooth pulp.
10. Add about 8 tablespoons of extra virgin olive oil with vinegar.
11. Pour over the vegetables and toss to coat in the basil oil. Discard the remaining basil leaves.
12. Add sliced garlic to the bowl with the fennel tops.
13. Give everything a good mix.
14. Serve and enjoy.

Grilled fillet steak with the creamiest white beans and leeks

Ingredients

- 4 x 200g of fillet steaks
- 4 leeks
- 1 lemon
- Sea salt
- 1 small bunch of fresh thyme
- 2 cloves garlic
- Olive oil
- 1 small wineglass white wine
- Freshly ground black pepper
- 500g of tinned butter beans
- Peppery extra virgin olive oil
- 1 small handful freshly picked parsley leaves
- 1 tablespoon of fat-free natural yoghurt

Directions

1. Firstly, sweat the leeks together with the thyme and garlic in a saucepan with a splash of olive oil over low heat for 20 minutes.
2. Raise the heat, then add the white wine.

3. Let the wine come to the boil.

4. After which add the beans with a splash of water, just to almost cover the beans.

5. Let simmer for 10 minutes until the beans are creamy.

6. Add the parsley together with the yoghurt and extra virgin olive oil.

7. Taste, and adjust the seasoning.

8. Heat a griddle pan until hot, season the steaks and pat with olive oil.

9. Grill a steak for 3 minutes on each side for medium-rare.

10. Remove from the grill on to a dish, let rest for 5 minutes.

11. Squeeze over some lemon juice and drizzle with extra virgin olive oil.

12. Carve the steaks into thick slices.

13. Divide the creamy beans between plates and place the steak on top

14. Serve and enjoy drizzled with resting juices.

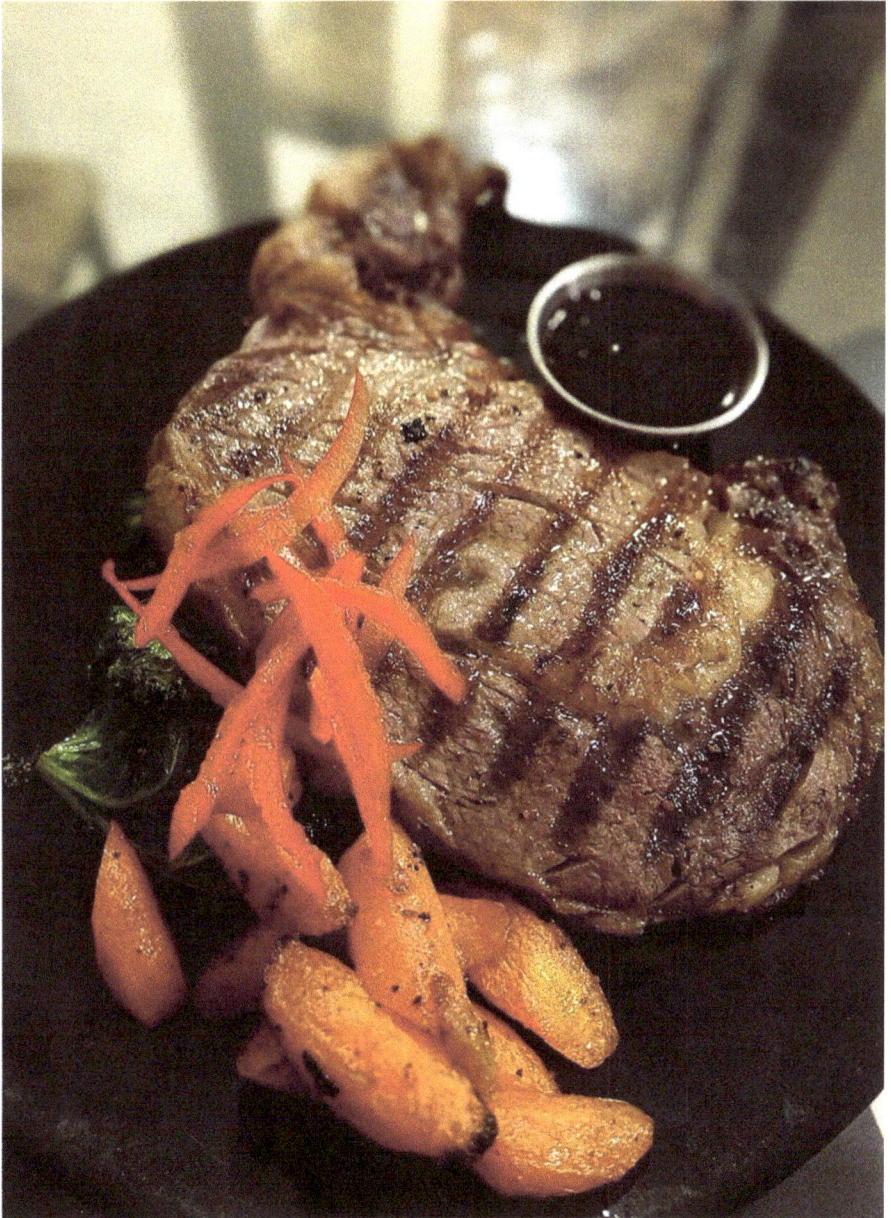

Spinach and ricotta cannelloni

Ingredients

- Parmesan cheese
- 150g of cannelloni
- Extra virgin olive oil
- 1 onion
- 2 x 125g of mozzarella balls
- 2 cloves of garlic
- 250g of ricotta
- 2 x 400g tins of quality plum tomatoes
- 400g of spinach
- 1 bay leaf
- ½ a bunch of fresh basil
- ¼ teaspoon of ground nutmeg
- ½ a lemon
- 1 large free-range egg

Directions

1. Preheat the oven to 350°F.
2. Put the spinach and a drizzle of olive oil in a large pan over a low heat.
3. Add the nutmeg, then season with sea salt and black pepper, cover, let sweat.

4. Dice the onion and squash the garlic.
5. In the same pan, heat a drizzle of olive oil and gently sweat the onion until soft.
6. Scrunch in the tomatoes, add the garlic and bay leaf.
7. Pick in a few basil leaves and grate in the zest of the lemon half.
8. Let simmer for 20 minutes until the sauce has thickened.
9. Season with salt and pepper.
10. Place the spinach on a board, chop.
11. Return the spinach to the liquid in the bowl.
12. Beat the egg and grate 2 teaspoons of Parmesan cheese.
13. Sit a piping bag in a jug, fold its edges over the rim, then spoon in the spinach mixture.
14. Spread the tomato sauce over the cannelloni.
15. Pick the remaining basil leaves and scatter most of them over the tomato sauce.
16. Slice the mozzarella and lay the slices on top.
17. Drizzle with extra virgin olive oil, season.
18. Place in the oven, let cook for 40 minutes or till the top is golden.
19. Remove from the oven and let stand for a few minutes.
20. Serve and enjoy.

Greens mac and cheese

Ingredients

- 450g of dried macaroni
- 1 large leek
- 30g of Parmesan cheese
- 3 cloves of garlic
- 400g of purple sprouting
- 1 liter of semi-skimmed milk
- 150g of mature Cheddar cheese
- 50g of flaked almonds
- 40g of unsalted butter
- ½ a bunch of fresh thyme
- 2 tablespoons of plain flour
- 100g of baby spinach

Directions

1. Preheat the oven to 350°F.
2. Place the sliced garlic, broccoli stalks, butter, thyme leaves, and leek in a large casserole pan over a medium heat, let cook for 15 minutes, stirring regularly.
3. Stir in the flour and milk, let simmer for 10 minutes, stirring regularly.

4. Cook the pasta in a large pan of boiling salted water for 5 minutes, drain.

5. Grate the Parmesan and most of the Cheddar into the sauce, mix.

6. Place into a blender, then add the spinach and whisk until smooth.

7. Season with sea salt and black pepper, stir through the pasta and broccoli florets.

8. Transfer to a baking dish, grate over the remaining Cheddar and scatter over the almonds.

9. Let bake for 30 minutes, or until bubbling.

10. Serve and enjoy.

Squash and spinach pasta rotolo

Ingredients

- 50g of feta cheese
- 1 red onion
- 20g of Parmesan cheese
- Olive oil
- 6 large fresh pasta sheets
- 1 teaspoon of dried thyme
- A few sprigs of fresh sage
- 500g of frozen spinach
- 1 butternut squash
- 1 whole nutmeg
- 4 cloves of garlic
- 1 x 700ml of jar of passata

Directions

1. Preheat the oven to 350°F.
2. Cook the squash whole on a roasting tray for around 1 hour 30 minutes.
3. Place chopped onions into a medium pan on a medium-low heat with olive oil, the thyme and a pinch of salt and pepper, let cook for 10 minutes, stirring occasionally.

4. Stir in the frozen spinach, cover with a lid and allow to slowly cook for another 15 minutes.
5. Season squash and spinach with sea salt, black pepper and a grating of nutmeg.
6. Place garlic in a shallow casserole pan on a medium heat with a splash of olive oil.
7. Fry for briefly until lightly golden.
8. Pour in the passata, with a splash of water to the empty jar, swirl around and pour into the pan.
9. Bring to the boil, then simmer for 3 minutes, season.
10. Lay out the pasta sheets facing lengthways.
11. Brush the pasta with water, then evenly divide and spread the squash over the sheets.
12. Sprinkle over the cooked spinach and crumble over the feta.
13. Roll up the sheets and cut each one into 4 chunks, then place side by side in the tomato sauce.
14. Finely grate over the Parmesan, then pick the sage leaves, toss in a little oil and scatter over the top.
15. Let bake for 40 minutes at the bottom of the oven until golden.
16. Serve and enjoy.

Creamed spinach

Ingredients

- 100g of cheddar cheese
- 2 onions
- 100g of unsalted butter
- 2 cloves of garlic
- 100g of plain flour
- Olive oil
- 2 teaspoons of dried oregano
- 250ml crème fraiche
- 1 whole nutmeg
- 1kg of frozen chopped spinach
- 100g of rolled oats

Directions

1. Preheat the oven to 350°F.
2. Place onions and garlic, oregano, and 2 tablespoons of olive oil in a large frying pan on a low heat.
3. Grate in half of the nutmeg, fry for 10 minutes, or until soft, stirring regularly.
4. Add the spinach, raise the heat to medium, let cook for 20 minutes, or until any liquid has evaporated.

5. Place butter with cheese flour, oats, and a pinch of sea salt and black pepper in a blender.
6. Blend into a crumble texture, then remove to a plate.
7. Put the cooked spinach mixture into the processor, then add the crème fraiche, blend for 1 minute.
8. Taste, and adjust the seasoning.
9. Place evenly into a baking dish.
10. Sprinkle over the crumble, let bake for around 45 minutes, or until golden.
11. Serve and enjoy.

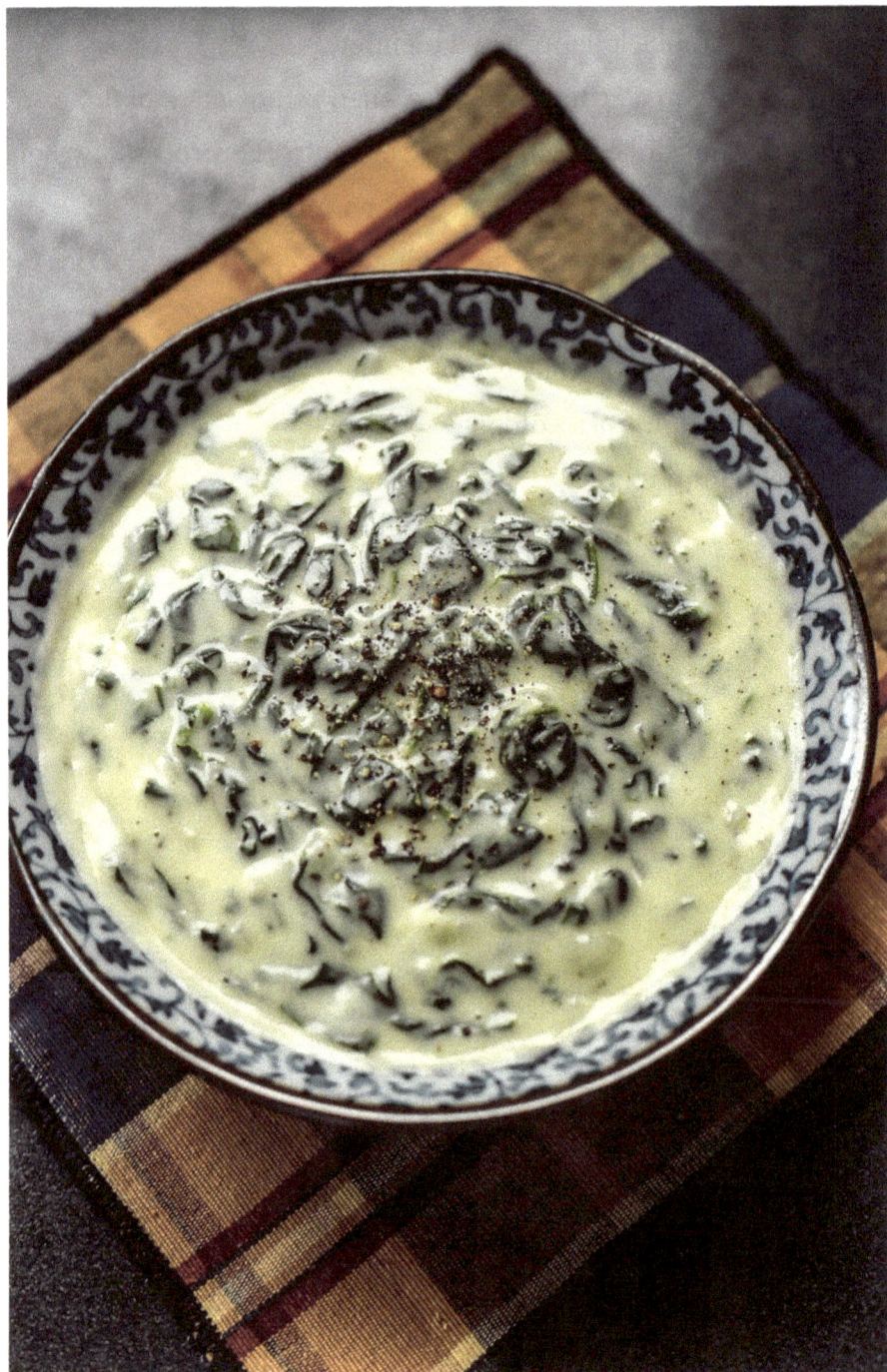

Speedy spinach curry

Ingredients

- 100g of paneer cheese
- 20g of unsalted cashew nuts
- 200g of baby spinach
- 1 onion
- Red wine vinegar
- 2 teaspoons of Rogan curry paste

Directions

1. Put a large frying pan on a medium-high heat.
2. Toast the cashew nuts as it heats up, shaking the pan occasionally until lightly golden.
3. Place the cashews into a pestle and mortar, returning the pan to the heat.
4. Place sliced onion in the hot pan with 1 tablespoon of olive oil and the curry paste.
5. Cook and stir for 8 minutes.
6. Add 1 tablespoon of red wine vinegar.
7. Let the vinegar cook away briefly, then, dice and add the paneer followed by the spinach.
8. Stir until the spinach is wilted, and liquid evaporated
9. Season with sea salt and black pepper.

10. Crush the cashew nuts and sprinkle over the top.

11. Serve and enjoy.

Smoky pancetta cod

Ingredients

- 1 x 250g sachet of cooked lentils
- 200g of spinach
- Red wine vinegar
- 8 rashers of smoked pancetta
- 2 x 150g of white fish fillets
- 2 sprigs of fresh rosemary

Directions

1. Lay out 4 rashers of pancetta, slightly overlapping them.
2. Place a piece of cod on top.
3. Then, generously season with black pepper.
4. Roll and wrap in the pancetta, and repeat.
5. Place in a large frying pan on a medium heat, let cook for 8 minutes, turning occasionally.
6. Add the rosemary for the last 2 minutes.
7. Remove the fish to a plate.
8. Toss the lentils into the pan with 1 tablespoon of red wine vinegar and push to one side to reheat for 1 minute.
9. Taste, and adjust the seasoning with sea salt and pepper
10. Sit the wrapped cod on top of the lentils with the rosemary.

11. Drizzle with 1 teaspoon of extra virgin olive oil.

12. Serve and enjoy.

Wilted spinach with yogurt and raisins

Ingredients

- 40g of raisins
- Extra virgin olive oil
- 1 small clove of garlic
- 300g of frozen spinach
- 500g of Greek yoghurt
- Sunflower oil

Directions

1. Place the spinach in a saucepan with a few tablespoons of water and cook over a medium heat briefly, or until defrosted.
2. Let cool.
3. Mix crushed garlic with the yoghurt, ¾ of a teaspoon of sea salt and a generous grind of black pepper.
4. Stir in the cooled spinach.
5. Heat sunflower oil in a small pan and fry the raisins for 2 minutes.
6. Scatter over the spinach and finish with a drizzle of extra virgin olive oil.

7. Serve and enjoy.

Spinach pici pasta

Ingredients

- Olive oil
- Extra virgin olive oil
- 4 cloves of garlic
- 50g of Parmesan cheese
- ½ teaspoon of dried red chili flakes
- 200g of baby spinach
- ½ a bunch of fresh basil
- 200g of baby courgettes
- 300g of plain flour
- 320g of ripe cherry tomatoes
- 50g of pine nuts

Directions

1. In a food processor, blend the spinach with flour until a ball of dough forms.
2. Tear off balls of dough, roll them out into long thin sausage shapes.
3. Cook the pici immediately, or leave them to dry out for a few hours.
4. Put a large pan of salted water to boil.

5. Put a large frying pan on a medium heat with 2 tablespoons of olive oil.
6. Add the sliced garlic with the chili flakes.
7. Add the courgettes with halved tomatoes, let cook for 5 minutes.
8. Stir in the pine nuts with a ladleful of boiling water. Cook over low heat.
9. Add the pici to the pan of boiling salted water for 8 5 minutes, and 8 minutes for dry one.
10. Drain, reserving a mugful of cooking water, toss through the vegetables.
11. Reserving the baby basil leaves, Stir into the pan the big chopped ones with grated Parmesan.
12. Divide between warm plates and serve with a few drips of extra virgin olive oil.
13. Enjoy.

Spinach lasagna

Ingredients

- 50g of plain flour
- 300g of fresh lasagna sheets
- 800ml of milk
- 100g of Parmesan cheese
- 1 fresh bay leaf
- 70g of unsalted butter
- 1 whole nutmeg
- 800g of spinach
- 200g of ricotta cheese

Directions

1. Preheat the oven ready to 375°F.
2. Melt the butter in a pan, then whisk in the flour.
3. Cook for 2 minutes, whisk in the milk till smooth.
4. Season with sea salt and freshly ground black pepper.
5. Add the bay leaf, let simmer for 5 minutes. Turn off the heat.
6. Remove the stalks from the spinach, then wilt with the remaining 20g butter in a covered pan, drain, let cool and squeeze out the liquid.

7. Mix chopped spinach with the ricotta and a ladleful of the white sauce and nutmeg. Season.

8. In a baking dish, layer the lasagna sheets with white sauce, spinach mixture, and a grating of Parmesan.

9. Finish with a layer of pasta topped with sauce and more Parmesan.

10. Let bake for 30 minutes, or till golden.

11. Serve and enjoy.

Monkfish with spinach and feta

Ingredients

- 50g of feta cheese
- 1 teaspoon of cumin seeds
- 200g of spinach
- ½ of a lemon
- 2 x 150g of monkfish fillets
- 2 sprigs of fresh thyme
- Olive oil

Directions

1. Crush and sprinkle the cumin seeds over the monkfish fillets.
2. Sprinkle the thyme leaves on top and season well.
3. Heat a little olive oil over a medium heat.
4. Add the fish and fry for 4 minutes on each side.
5. Bring a large pan of salted water to the boil.
6. Then, blanch the spinach for about 3 minutes.
7. Drain and drizzle with oil.
8. Serve and enjoy with the monkfish, sprinkled with the feta.

Spring pie

Ingredients

- 1 lemon
- Olive oil
- 1 x 270g packet of filo pastry
- 1 teaspoon of mustard powder
- 3 medium leeks
- 200ml of milk
- 200g of baby spinach
- 6 rashers of smoked streaky bacon
- ½ a bunch of fresh chives
- 6 large free-range eggs

Directions

1. Start by preheating the oven ready to 350°F.
2. Grease the baking dish with olive oil.
3. Cover the baking dish with a layer of pastry, letting the edges overhang slightly.
4. Brush with bit of olive oil.
5. Add another layer of pastry, repeating until all the pastry is done
6. Boil the kettle, then place the spinach in a colander.
7. Pour over the hot water to wilt.

8. Push the spinach down with the back of a spoon, then, when it's cool enough to handle, squeeze out any excess water.

9. Place the spinach on a board and roughly chop, then place in a large bowl and set aside.

10. Put the grill on high and grill the bacon till crisp, let cool.

11. Whisk the eggs in a large bowl with a pinch of sea salt and black pepper.

12. Then, whisk in the milk together with the mustard powder, chives, and grate in the lemon zest.

13. Crumble the cooled bacon into the spinach.

14. Add the leeks. Mix and scatter into the filo pastry case.

15. Pour over the egg mixture and place the dish on the bottom of the oven.

16. Let bake for 40 minutes.

17. Let cool for 20 minutes.

18. Serve sliced and enjoy with a crisp green salad.

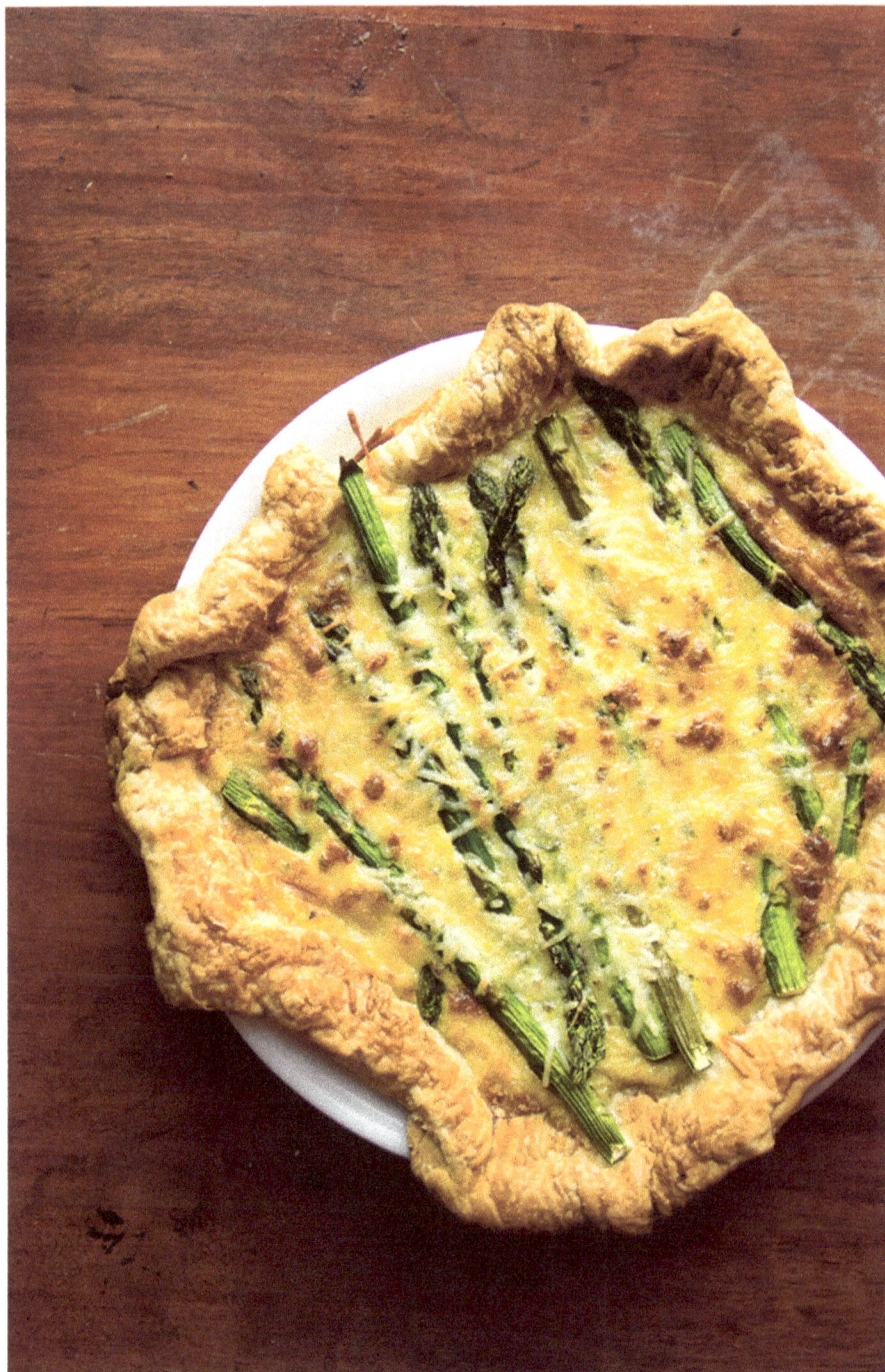

Curried cauliflower, potatoes, chickpeas, and spinach

Ingredients

- 1 teaspoon of ground cumin
- 1 cauliflower
- 1 teaspoon of mustard seeds
- 800g of potatoes
- 1 teaspoon of ground ginger
- 2 cloves of garlic
- Natural yoghurt
- 1 teaspoon of ground coriander
- 1 onion
- 1 teaspoon of curry powder
- 1 long green chili
- 2 tablespoons of olive oil
- 2 tablespoons of unsalted butter
- 1 lime
- 1 teaspoon of turmeric
- 1 x 400g tin of chickpeas
- 250g of baby spinach

Directions

1. Cook separated cauliflower in boiling salted water for 5 minutes, drain, reserve some of its cooking water.
2. Roughly chop the potatoes and cook in boiling salted water for 10 minutes, drain excess water.
3. Heat the olive oil and butter in a large frying pan, then sauté the garlic with the onion and chili till softened over low heat.
4. Stir in all the spices.
5. Season, let cook briefly.
6. Add the cooked cauliflower, potatoes, and reserved cooking water.
7. Let simmer over low heat for 10 minutes.
8. Drain and add the chickpeas with the spinach.
9. Cook, stirring, until the spinach wilts.
10. Then, transfer to a serving bowl.
11. Serve and enjoy with a dollop of yoghurt and a squeeze of lime juice.

Healthy greens box

Ingredients

- 1 heaped teaspoon harissa
- ½ a small head of broccoli
- 50g of feta cheese
- 1 handful of mixed seeds
- 1 handful of baby spinach
- ½ a small bunch of fresh mint
- Olive oil
- 80g of couscous
- 1 lemon
- 1 pinch of ground cumin

Directions

1. Cook the chopped broccoli in boiling water for 4 minutes.
2. Plunge into cold water to stop it cooking, then shake off excess water, place on a chopping board with the spinach.
3. Pick over a few large mint leaves and throw on a good pinch of salt and pepper.
4. Chop until finely chopped.
5. Scrape these straight into your lunchbox, pour the uncooked couscous on top and gently sit a lemon half in it.

6. Toast the seeds in a dry frying pan, then mix with the cumin and wrap in Clingfilm.

7. Add the juice from the remaining lemon half with a good swig of olive oil, harissa, and a few small mint leaves, then crumble in the feta in a small jar. Mix well.

8. Seal and place in the lunch box.

9. Boil the kettle when it is time to feast.

10. Take the lemon, seeds and jar from your lunchbox, then pour in boiling water to just cover the couscous.

11. Cover, and wait for 10 minutes until the water is absorbed.

12. Serve and enjoy.

Brilliant broccoli

Ingredients

- A small knob of unsalted butter
- 1 large head of broccoli
- Sea salt
- Freshly ground black pepper

Directions

1. Fill a large pan with slightly salted water, bring to the boil over a high heat.
2. Once boiling, lower the broccoli into the water using a slotted spoon.
3. Let cook for 4 minutes.
4. Drain in a colander, steam dry for a minute.
5. Place back into the pan, sprinkle with a tiny pinch of salt and pepper.
6. Add the butter tossing to coat.
7. Serve and enjoy.

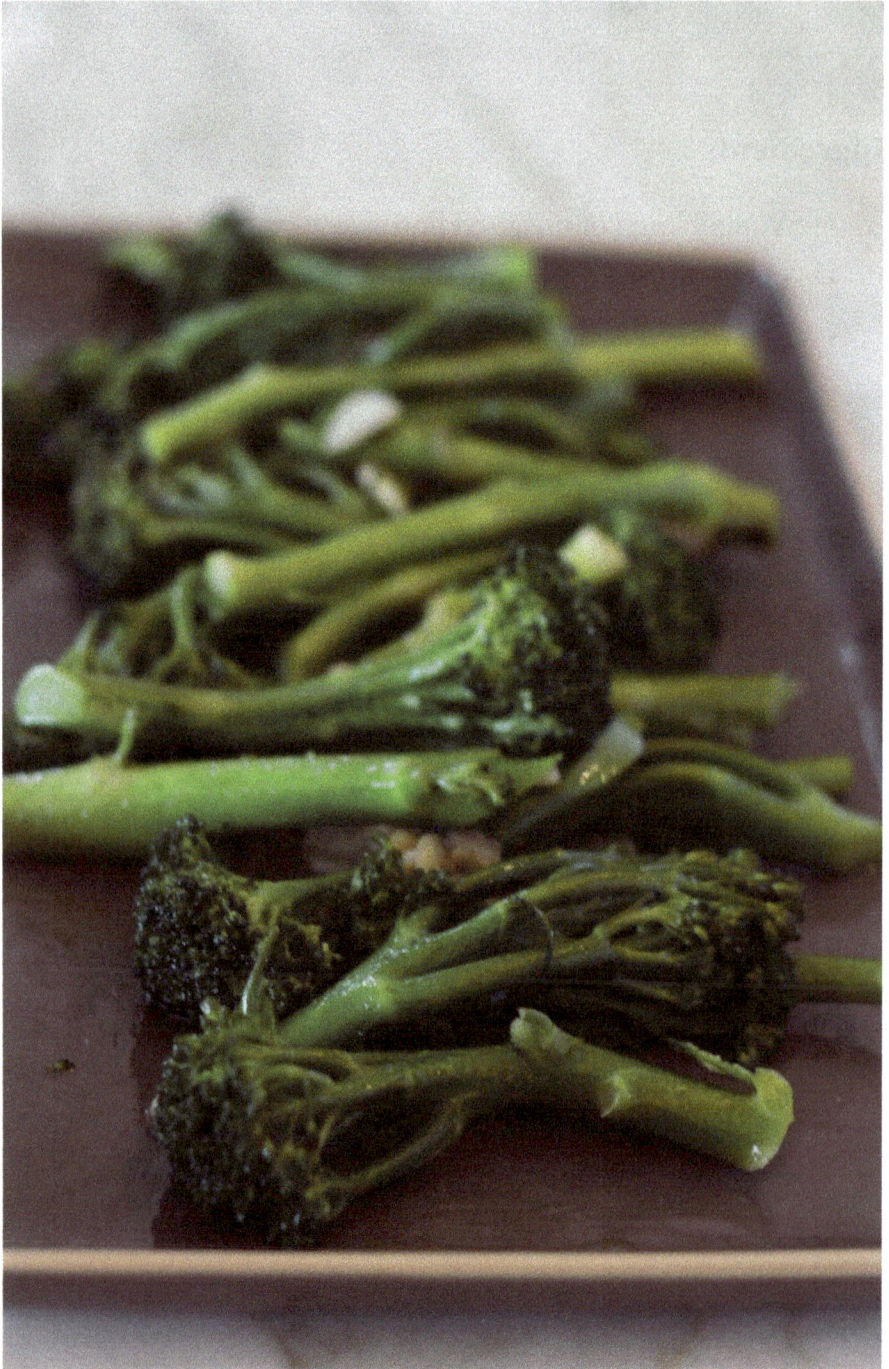

Steamed vegetables with flavored butters

Ingredients

- 500g of baby turnips
- 1 pinch of cumin seeds
- 350g of broccoli, cut into florets
- 1 tablespoon of fresh thyme
- Unsalted butter
- 1 clove garlic, chopped
- 450g of carrots, cut into thick strips
- 1 pinch of sugar
- ¼ orange, finely grated zest of
- ½ tablespoon of chopped fresh rosemary
- 3 anchovy fillets, chopped
- 2 sun-dried tomatoes in oil, drained and finely chopped
- ½ lemon
- 350g of mange tout, trimmed
- ½ red chili, deseeded and finely chopped

Directions

1. Pound the garlic together with the chili and sun-dried tomatoes in a pestle and mortar to a paste.

2. Add seasoning and the butter, pound well.

3. Dollop onto a sheet of greaseproof paper and roll into a cylinder, twisting the ends.

4. Place in the freezer to firm up.

5. Then, pound the sugar together with the zest, cumin seeds, and thyme.

6. Combine the broccoli, the rosemary, and anchovies, pound.

7. Mix the lemon juice and zest.

8. Then add the seasoning and butter, pound and roll into Christmas cracker shapes, as before.

9. Place the vegetables in a 2-layer steamer. Make sure carrots are closer to the heat, turnips, broccoli florets, then mange tout.

10. Steam for 10 minutes.

11. Serve and enjoy each vegetable with circles of flavored butter melted over the top.

Broccoli salad

Ingredients

- 6 tablespoons of extra virgin olive oil
- 2 large heads of broccoli
- 2 teaspoons of Dijon mustard
- 6 rashers of smoked streaky bacon
- 3 firm red tomatoes
- 2 tablespoons of white wine vinegar
- Olive oil
- ½ a bunch of fresh chives
- ½ a clove of garlic

Directions

1. Blanch the broccoli florets and sliced stalks quickly in boiling salted water for 60 seconds.
2. Drain in a colander, steam dry.
3. Transfer to a serving dish once totally dry.
4. Then, fry the sliced bacon on a medium heat with a small splash of olive oil until crisp and golden.
5. Spoon most of the bacon bits over the broccoli.
6. Pour into a mixing bowl, then grate in the garlic, adding the Dijon mustard, extra virgin olive oil, white wine vinegar.

7. Season with sea salt and black pepper, and whisk.
8. Chop the chives, reserving the flowers.
9. Add to the broccoli and bacon bits.
10. Serve and enjoy.

Mango, spinach, and pine nuts recipe

Ingredients

- ½ of a ripe mango
- 1 large handful of baby spinach
- 2 tablespoons of Greek yoghurt
- 1 tablespoon of pine nuts

Directions

1. Prepare the mangoes into bite-sized chunks.
2. Place in a blender.
3. Add the yoghurt together with the spinach and pine nuts, blend to a purée.
4. Adjust the thickness with water to loosen.
5. Serve and enjoy chilled.

Sag paneer

Ingredients

- freshly ground black pepper
- groundnut oil
- 1 onion
- 1.5 liters of whole milk
- 2 cloves of garlic
- 600g of frozen spinach
- 5cm piece of ginger
- 1 lemon
- sea salt
- 1 teaspoon of cumin seeds
- 2 teaspoons of Garam masala
- 50ml of single cream
- ½ teaspoon of ground turmeric
- 1 ripe tomato

Directions

1. Line a sieve with a large piece of muslin and place over a bowl.
2. Heat the milk in a large heavy-based pan over a medium heat.
3. Bring to the boil, then reduce the heat to a gentle simmer.

4. Add 4 tablespoons of lemon juice, then pour the mixture into the sieve. Place under cold running water, gather up the muslin and squeeze out the excess moisture.

5. Place in the fridge for 1 hour 30 minutes, then cut the paneer into chunks.

6. Drizzle olive oil into a large non-stick frying pan over a medium heat, place in the paneer and fry for 5 minutes, stirring frequently. Drain.

7. Return the pan to a medium-low heat, add cumin seeds and onion, fry for 8 minute, or until softened.

8. Stir in the garlic with ginger, Garam masala, chopped tomatoes, and turmeric. Cook for 10 minutes, stirring occasionally.

9. Stir in the frozen spinach, then add the cream, paneer and a splash of boiling water.

10. Lower the heat, let cook for 5 minutes uncovered, or until reduced to a creamy consistency.

11. Season with sea salt and black pepper.

12. Serve and enjoy.

Chickpea and spiced spinach smash with sweet potato

Ingredients

- 1 x 400g tin of chickpeas in water
- 1 teaspoon of olive oil
- 1 small onion
- 200g of fresh spinach
- 1 clove of garlic
- 1 large sweet potato
- ½ teaspoon of garam masala
- ½ teaspoon of turmeric

Directions

1. Cook the sweet potato in boiling water until tender, drain and mash.
2. Heat the oil in a medium pan over low heat.
3. Add the onion and fry for 8 minutes.
4. Add the garlic together with the turmeric and garam masala, cook for 3 minutes.
5. Drain the chickpeas, add to the pan along with the spinach.

6. Cover, let cook for 10 minutes, or until the spinach has wilted.
7. Mash the mixture with until fairly smooth with some soft lumps, let cool.
8. Serve the cooled chickpea smash with the mashed sweet potato.
9. Enjoy.

Beetroot and avocado Mediterranean Sea diet recipes

Whereas beetroots help to improve the general blood supply in the body, avocados are quite significant in nourishing the human skin among other health benefits.

Like other recipe, the beetroot and avocado recipes can be accompanying by other plants for salad or whole meal.

Avocados are quite plenty in most parts of the world, and so beetroot that are scarce in some parts of Africa.

The beetroot and avocado recipes include but following.

Gravadlax recipe

Ingredients

- 50g of fresh grated horseradish
- 1 big bunch of fresh dill
- 200g of raw beets
- 1 lemon
- 100g of rock salt
- 50g of demerara sugar
- 1 x 700g side of salmon
- 50ml of vodka

Directions

1. Place the beets in a food processor together with sugar, vodka, salt, and dill.
2. Grate in the lemon zest and add horseradish, blend to combine.
3. Rub bit of the mixture on to the salmon skin, then put on a large tray, skin side down, cover completely with the mixture.
4. Cover the tray tightly with Clingfilm with a weight on top.
5. Place into the fridge for 36 hours.
6. Once cured, unwrap the fish, pour the juices down the sink and rub salty topping.

7. Pat the fillet dry, then tightly wrap in Clingfilm. Keep in the fridge until needed.
8. Slice and enjoy.

Beetroot, carrot, and orange salad

Ingredients

- ½ a bunch of fresh coriander
- Olive oil
- 2 oranges
- 500g of raw beetroot
- 1 tablespoon of sesame seeds
- 750g of carrots
- Extra virgin olive oil

Directions

1. Preheat the oven to 400ºF.
2. Parboil the carrots in a large pan of boiling salted water for 5 minutes.
3. Move to a colander using a slotted spoon.
4. Place in the beets and parboil for 5 minutes, then drain.
5. Transfer the carrots with the beets to a large roasting tin, then, drizzle with olive oil.
6. Season with sea salt and black pepper.
7. Let roast for 40 minutes, or until shiny, shake the tray occasionally.

8. Toast the sesame seeds over low heat until golden, tossing regularly.

9. Let cool, toss with the orange zest and segments, extra virgin olive oil.

10. Arrange over a large platter, scatter over the toasted sesame seeds and coriander leaves.

11. Serve and enjoy.

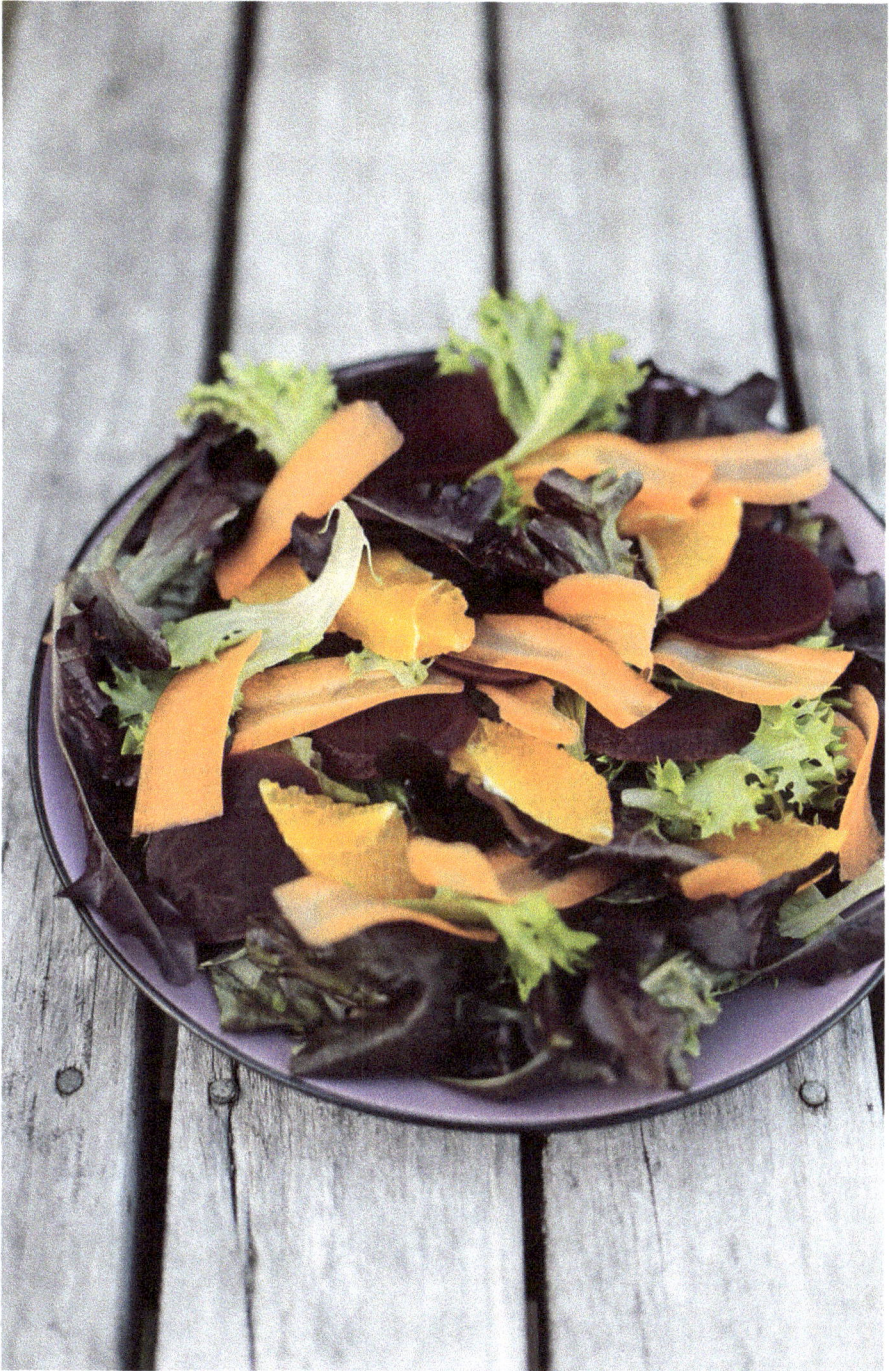

Potato rosti with beetroot horseradish

Ingredients

- 1½ teaspoons of cumin seeds
- 2 medium beetroots
- ½ a red onion
- 2 tablespoons of creamed horseradish
- 1 clove of garlic
- 2 large potatoes
- 3 tablespoons of vegetable oil

Directions

1. Coarsely grate and squeeze out excess liquid from the potatoes.
2. Then, combine the potatoes together with the onion, toasted cumin, and garlic in a large bowl, season.
3. Shape into 4 patties with your hands.
4. Heat olive oil in a pan.
5. Fry the rosti over a medium-low heat for 10 minutes on each side, turning carefully.
6. Combine the grated beetroot with horseradish in a bowl and serve on top of the rosti.
7. Enjoy.

Beetroot nicoise salad

Ingredients

- 1 bunch of fresh mixed soft herbs
- 2 small cos lettuce
- 4 slices of sourdough bread
- 12 quail eggs
- 500g of raw mixed baby beetroots
- 1 tablespoon of red wine vinegar
- 2 teaspoons of Dijon mustard
- 1 tablespoon of baby capers
- 4 salted anchovy fillets
- 4 tablespoons of extra virgin olive oil
- 150g of fine French beans
- 100g of ripe cherry tomatoes

Directions

1. Boil water in large pans.
2. Place beetroots into one of the pans, keeping some for later, let boil for 10 minutes. Slice the reserved beets.
3. Whisking extra virgin olive oil with vinegar, mustard, and capers.
4. Season with sea salt and black pepper.
5. Drain the beetroots in a colander and steam dry.

6. Peel the skin and slice any larger beetroots in half.
7. Transfer the beetroots to a bowl, drizzle over half the dressing, toss to coat.
8. In the other pan, add the quail eggs with the French beans, let simmer for 4 minutes, then drain.
9. Add the flavoring herbs to the leftover dressing, place into a salad bowl.
10. Layer up the tomatoes in the salad bowl with the lettuce and anchovies, drizzle over the dressing.
11. Next, tumble in the cooked and raw beetroots with the eggs and green beans.
12. Scatter over the remaining herbs.
13. Serve and enjoy with the sourdough.

Beetroot crisp with coriander hummus

Ingredients

- 1 teaspoon of smoked paprika
- 250g of large beetroot
- 1 lemon
- 3 sprigs of fresh thyme
- 2 tablespoons of tahini
- Olive oil
- Extra virgin olive oil
- 2 cloves of garlic
- 1 x 400g tin of chickpeas
- 50g of coriander leaves

Directions

1. Preheat your oven ready to 400°F.
2. Place sliced beetroots in a bowl. Toss in the thyme leaves with bit of olive oil.
3. Spread on a lined baking trays, let roast for 15 minutes, let cool.
4. In a blender, crush the garlic, and pour in the chickpeas with their juices.

5. Add the remaining ingredients with bit of extra virgin olive oil, blend until smooth.

6. Season, drizzle with extra virgin olive oil in a bowl.

7. Serve and enjoy.

Roasted beetroot, red onion, and watercress salad

Ingredients

- 5 tablespoons of olive oil
- 3 tablespoons of baby caper
- 2 x 600g bunches of beetroot
- 4 red onions
- 125ml of white wine
- A few sprigs of fresh dill
- 4 tablespoons of extra virgin olive oil
- A few sprigs of fresh mint leaves
- 4 cloves of garlic
- A few sprigs of parsley leaves
- 2 x 75g bags of watercress
- 3 tablespoons of balsamic vinegar
- 1 tablespoon of Dijon mustard

Directions

1. Preheat the oven to 340°F.
2. Place sliced beetroots in a baking tin with 2 tablespoons of olive oil, fill the tin with water.
3. Cover the dish with tin foil, let bake for 1 hour.

4. Remove the beets from the tin, let cool.
5. Toss the onion wedges in 2 tablespoons of the olive oil on the baking tray, season.
6. Add to the oven, let roast for about 30 minutes.
7. Remove, let cool.
8. Rub the off the beetroot skins, cut into wedges.
9. Blanch the beetroot stalks and leaves in a pan of boiling salted water for 2 minutes, drain.
10. Heat the remaining tablespoon of oil in a pan over a high heat.
11. Then, add the beetroot stalks and garlic and fry until the garlic is golden.
12. Lower the heat to medium, pour in the wine, let cook for 10 minutes.
13. Add the beetroot leaves, season, cook until wilted.
14. Whisk the vinegar into the mustard, then stir in the olive oil and season to taste.
15. In a large serving bowl, gently toss the roasted beetroot and red onions with the stalk mixture, chopped herbs, capers and vinaigrette, then mix with the watercress.
16. Serve and enjoy.

Harvest salad

Ingredients

- 2 tablespoon of red wine vinegar
- 6 tablespoons of extra virgin olive oil
- 6 small beetroots
- 1 red onion
- 2 bulbs of fennel
- 1 teaspoon of Dijon mustard
- Olive oil
- 2 teaspoons of coriander seeds
- ½ a bunch of fresh mint
- 1 acorn squash
- ½ a bunch of fresh flat-leaf parsley
- 1 pomegranate
- 150g of feta cheese

Directions

1. Preheat the oven ready to 380°F.
2. Lay cut squash pieces, beetroots, fennel wedges and sliced onions in a roasting tray.
3. Drizzle with a little olive oil.
4. Pound the coriander seeds with a good pinch each of sea salt and black pepper.

5. Sprinkle over the vegetables on the tray, toss to coat.

6. Let roast for about 40 minutes, shaking halfway through. Let cool slightly.

7. The, combine the vinegar together with the extra virgin olive oil, mustard, and seasoning in a small jug. Mix well.

8. Dress the roasted veg while still warm so they soak up all the dressing.

9. Sprinkle over the herb leaves, and reserved fennel tops.

10. Add the pomegranate to the vegetables. Crumble over the feta.

11. Serve and enjoy.

Roasted beetroot toast

Ingredients

- 4 slices of sourdough
- A few fresh chives
- 4 tablespoons of red wine vinegar
- 4 raw beetroots
- 5 sprigs of fresh thyme
- 2 tablespoons of creamed horseradish

Directions

1. Preheat the oven to 350°F.
2. Place wedges of beetroot in a roasting tray.
3. Add the vinegar together with the thyme and 4 tablespoons of water, toss to coat.
4. Cover with tin foil, then let roast for 45 minutes.
5. Toast the bread and spread with the horseradish topping with the roasted beetroot.
6. Serve and enjoy.

Gluten-free spinach and ricotta roulade

Ingredients

- Olive oil
- 1 lemon
- 1 pinch of chili flakes
- 2 cloves of garlic
- 60g of whole blanched almonds
- 1 fresh red chili
- 1 kg butternut squash
- 1 teaspoon of fennel seeds
- 6 large free-range eggs
- 100g of crumbly goat's cheese
- 80g of Parmesan cheese
- 150g of ricotta cheese
- 60g of gluten-free plain flour
- 1 whole nutmeg
- 300g of baby spinach

Directions

1. Preheat the oven to 375ºF.
2. Line a shallow baking tin with greaseproof paper.

3. Place prepared squash into a large roasting tray with a splash of olive oil, chili flakes, and bit of pinch of salt and pepper. Toss to coat.

4. Add garlic cloves, then place in the hot oven for 1 hour.

5. Place a frying pan over a medium heat with almonds, fennel seeds, and a pinch of salt.

6. Let cook for 4 minutes, or until golden. Bash in a mortar.

7. Remove from oven, then scoop the flesh and garlic into a food processor and discard the skin. Blend till smooth.

8. Separate the egg yolks from the whites into two large bowls.

9. Grate the Parmesan over the yolks, stir in the squash purée together with the flour, nutmeg, and a pinch of salt and pepper.

10. Fold into the squash mixture.

11. Transfer to the lined tin, spreading evenly.

12. Let bake for 15 minutes, or until set.

13. Heat a splash of olive oil over a medium heat, add spinach, let cook for 2 minutes until wilted.

14. Turn out the roulade onto a large piece of greaseproof paper.

15. Crumble the goat's cheese into a bowl, add the ricotta together with the lemon zest and juice.

16. Add chili, stir.

17. Season with sea salt and black pepper.

18. Spread the mixture over the sponge, scatter over the spinach and 1/3 of the almonds.
19. Roll up the sponge, using the greaseproof paper.
20. Serve and enjoy.

Giant vegetable rosti

Ingredients

- 100g of baby spinach
- 600g of potatoes
- 3 large carrots
- Olive oil
- 4 large free-range eggs
- 100g of frozen peas
- ½ teaspoon of Dijon mustard
- 50g of feta cheese
- ½ of a lemon
- Extra virgin olive oil

Directions

1. Preheat the oven to 350°F.
2. Coarsely grate potatoes and carrots in a food processor.
3. Add a good pinch of sea salt, toss, let rest for 5 minutes.
4. Combine the mustard together with a squeeze of lemon juice, extra virgin olive oil, and a little pinch of salt and black pepper in a medium bowl.
5. Drizzle olive oil into a large bowl.
6. Add a good pinch of pepper.

7. Then, squeeze the potato and carrot mixture, then sprinkle into the bowl.

8. Toss in the oil with the pepper until mixed.

9. Scatter over a large oiled baking tray.

10. Roast for 35 minutes or so, until golden on top.

11. In a large pan of salted boiling water, blanch the peas for a minute.

12. Then, add to the bowl of dressing and pile the spinach on top.

13. Crack in the eggs when the rosti is about to get ready, poach and remove.

14. Serve the rosti with the eggs on top.

15. Serve and enjoy.

Perfect braised spinach

Ingredients

- 10g of butter
- 400g of spinach
- 1 grating nutmeg
- ½ lemon, juice

Directions

1. Place little butter, nutmeg grating, spinach, and a tiny squeeze of lemon juice into a pan.
2. Cover, and cook with steam.
3. Let the spinach sit for a minute.
4. Serve and enjoy.

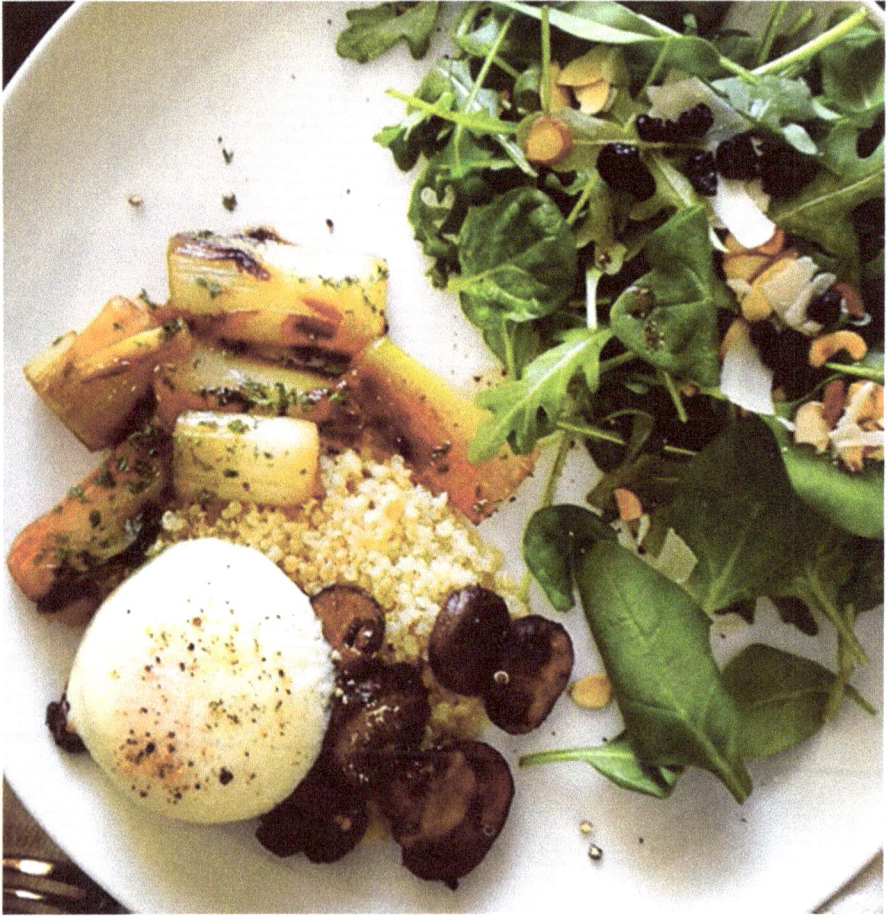

Roast trout with spinach, sage, and prosciutto

Ingredients

- 410g of tinned cannellini beans
- 75g of ground almonds
- 2 handfuls of dried apricots, chopped
- 4 large slices quality prosciutto
- 2 large sprigs fresh sage
- 600g of spinach
- Olive oil
- 8 x 120g of trout fillets
- 410g of tinned chickpeas
- 1 clove garlic, crushed
- Fresh nutmeg, grated

Directions

1. Preheat the oven to 400ºF.
2. Season the trout with salt and pepper, dust in the ground almonds.
3. Lay 4 of the fillets on a board, skin-side down.
4. Mix apricot and ½ of the sage together, then lay in a line along the tops of the 4 fillets.

5. Top with the remaining fillets, skin-side up, matching heads and tails with the 4 below.

6. Overlap the remaining sage along the length of each trout sandwich.

7. Cut 4 x 20cm lengths of string and lay them parallel to each other on a work surface.

8. Lay 1 of the trout sandwiches across the lengths of string and tie them all up.

9. Repeat with the rest.

10. Heat a large saucepan.

11. Add a large splash of oil and gently fry the garlic until softened.

12. Add the spinach, seasoning with salt and pepper and the grated nutmeg.

13. Spread the spinach out in a roasting tray, and mix with the pulses.

14. Lay the prosciutto slices over the bean mixture.

15. Drizzle with olive oil, bake for 20 minutes until the prosciutto is crispy.

Cumberland roast chicken

Ingredients

- 1 x 1.5kg of whole chicken
- 1.2 kg potatoes
- 3 Cumberland sausages
- 1 pear
- 2 parsnips
- 2 leeks
- 85g of watercress
- Olive oil
- ½ bunch of sage

Directions

1. Preheat the oven to 360°F.
2. Place potatoes, parsnips, and leeks in a roasting tray, then toss with 2 tablespoons of olive oil, a pinch of sea salt and black pepper and the sage leaves.
3. Squeeze the sausage meat out of the skins, make sure to scrunch together.
4. Poke half the sausage meat into each side, smooth well.
5. Secure the skin with a cocktail stick.
6. Rub the chicken with a pinch of salt and pepper and 1 tablespoon of oil.

7. Stuff the sage stalks into the chicken cavity.

8. Place the chicken directly on the bars of the oven with the tray of vegetables underneath, let roast until everything is golden.

9. Sprinkle the reserved sage leaves over the tray of vegetables.

10. Slice the pear, and toss with the watercress.

11. Sit the chicken on the vegetables.

12. Serve and enjoy.

Sausage and mash pie

Ingredients

- 6 Cumberland
- 4 tablespoons of plain flour
- Olive oil
- 3 teaspoons of English mustard
- 2 large leeks
- 1.2kg of potatoes
- ½ a bunch of thyme
- 2 eating apples
- 600ml of semi-skimmed milk

Directions

1. Preheat the oven to 400°F.
2. Cook chopped potatoes in a large pan of salted boiling water for 15 minutes.
3. In a large non-stick casserole pan, brown the sausages on a medium heat, tossing regularly.
4. Add 1 tablespoon of olive oil with the leek.
5. Remove the sausages once golden, place in the leek with apple, thyme, and splash of water.
6. Season with sea salt and black pepper, cook for 20 minutes, covered, stirring occasionally.

7. Drain the potatoes, and mash with half of the flour.
8. Lightly rub a baking dish with oil.
9. Spread 2/3 of the mash evenly across the base and sides of the dish.
10. Stir the remaining flour into the leeks, together with the milk, and mustard.
11. Simmer for 5 minutes.
12. Stir sausages into the pan with any juices, then evenly spoon into the mash-lined dish.
13. Press the remaining mash on to a sheet of greaseproof paper until bigger than the dish, then flip over the top of the dish, crimp the edges with a fork to seal.
14. Poke the reserved sausage slices into the top, brush with 1 tablespoon of oil.
15. Let bake for 40 minutes.
16. Serve and enjoy.

Sweet leek carbonara

Ingredients

- Olive oil
- 2 large leeks
- 4 cloves of garlic
- 50g of Parmesan or pecorino cheese
- 1 large free-range egg
- 4 sprigs of fresh thyme
- 1 knob of unsalted butter
- 300g of dried spaghetti

Directions

1. Combine the leek and garlic in a large casserole pan over medium heat with the butter and 1 tablespoon of olive oil.
2. When sizzling, stir in the leeks and water, let simmer, covered over a low heat for 40 minutes, stirring occasionally.
3. Season with sea salt and black pepper.
4. Then, cook the pasta in a large pan of boiling salted water according to the packet Directions.
5. Drain, reserving some pasta cooking water.
6. Toss the drained pasta into the leek pan, then remove from the heat.

7. Hold on for 2 minutes to let cool briefly, then beat in eggs with cheese, toss.
8. Serve and enjoy with white wine.

Quiche leekraine

Ingredients

- 250ml of milk
- 300g of leeks
- 1 x 20cm precooked pastry case
- Olive oil
- 3 large eggs
- 3 slices of smoked streaky bacon
- Green salad
- 75g of Cheddar cheese

Directions

1. Preheat the oven to 360°F.
2. Sauté the leek with a splash of oil until sticky.
3. Fry the chopped bacon in a separate pan until golden.
4. Whisk the eggs and stir the cheese in the cheese, milk, leeks, bacon, and pinch of seasoning.
5. Place the pastry case onto a baking sheet.
6. Pour the mixture into the case.
7. Let bake for 30 minutes.
8. Serve and enjoy with a mixed green salad.

Ham and peas

Ingredients

- ½ a bunch of fresh curly parsley
- 3 ham hocks
- 400g of frozen peas
- 100g of pearl barley
- 2 leeks
- 1 stick of celery
- 1 heaped tablespoon of mint sauce
- 3 carrots
- Olive oil
- 2 fresh bay leaves
- 1 liter of organic chicken stock

Directions

1. Soak the ham hocks in cold water overnight.
2. Drain, refill with fresh cold water and bring to the boil.
3. Discard the salty water, rinse the hocks, repeat once again.
4. Combine the leeks with the celery, and carrots in a food processor.
5. Add the vegetables to a pan with olive oil, bay leaves, a pinch of sea salt and black pepper.

6. Sweat over a medium heat for 15 minutes, stirring occasionally.
7. Add the drained ham hocks, pearl barley, and chicken stock.
8. Let boil, then cook over a medium-low heat for 3 hours when covered.
9. Transfer the ham hocks to a clean board, remove all the fat and bones.
10. Shred the meat then return it to the broth.
11. Raise the heat, add the peas.
12. Cook until tender, then finely chop and stir in the parsley with the mint sauce.
13. Serve and enjoy with bread.

Cheesy leeks

Ingredients

- 50g of Parmesan cheese
- 6 large leeks
- 1 knob of unsalted butter
- 2 cloves of garlic
- 100g of Cheddar cheese
- 100g of brie
- 5 sprigs of fresh thyme
- Olive oil
- 100ml of single cream

Directions

1. Preheat the oven to 350ºF.
2. Over a medium heat, place a large casserole pan
3. Drizzle with bit of oil, butter, thyme leaves, and garlic.
4. Cook until bubbling, fry, then stir in the leeks.
5. Stir the rest of the ingredients into the leeks, with grated Cheddar and Parmesan, and brie, then place in the oven cook for 45 minutes uncovered.
6. Season, then spoon it all into a dish.
7. Stir in the cream and splash of water.
8. Grate over the Cheddar and Parmesan.

9. Pull the brie into parts, place on top.
10. Place in the oven for 15 minutes.
11. Serve and enjoy.

Crostini of smoked salmon butter and poached leeks

Ingredients

- 5 sprigs of fresh chervil
- 160g of unsalted butter
- 200ml of white wine
- 10 baby leeks
- 130g of smoked salmon
- 60g of unsalted butter
- 60ml of olive oil
- 20ml of fresh lemon juice
- 2 fresh bay leaves
- 12 slices of ciabatta
- 3 sprigs of fresh thyme
- 200ml of quality fish stock
- 40g of salted baby capers

Directions

1. Combine the butter with smoked salmon, and lemon juice in a food processor, blend until smooth.
2. Season and set aside.

3. Combine butter, olive oil, bay leaves, and thyme to a wide, shallow saucepan over a medium-low heat, let simmer.
4. Add the leeks, let cook for 10 minutes, until golden.
5. Pour in the stock with the wine, cover with a baking paper, let cook for 15 minutes.
6. Remove from the heat and rest the leeks in the liquid.
7. Put the capers in a small saucepan with enough olive oil to cover.
8. Place over a high heat, fry until the capers crisp up.
9. Transfer the capers to a plate lined with kitchen paper using a slotted spoon.
10. Heat a griddle pan over medium high heat.
11. Brush the ciabatta with olive oil and toast until golden.
12. Spread the toasted ciabatta generously with the smoked salmon butter.
13. Serve and enjoy topped with the leeks and fried capers

Ham and leek quiche

Ingredients

- 300ml of semi-skimmed milk
- 2 leeks
- 1 shallot
- 8 sprigs of fresh thyme
- 4 sheets of filo pastry
- 75g of mature Cheddar
- 60g of smoked ham
- 3 large eggs
- 10g of unsalted butter
- 200g of sprouting broccoli
- 1 tablespoon of olive oil

Directions

1. Preheat the oven to 350°F.
2. Melt butter in a pan, then sauté the leeks with the shallot and half the thyme leaves for 5 minutes.
3. Blanch the broccoli in boiling salted water for about 3 minutes. Drain.
4. Brush a quiche tin with a little of the olive oil, drape with a layer of filo pastry, leaving some overhanging.
5. Brush the filo with a little more oil.

6. Scatter over some of the remaining thyme leaves and layer another piece of filo on top. Repeat layering the oil, thyme and filo until you have a fully lined quiche base.

7. Bake the case for 5 minutes.

8. Stir the broccoli together with the smoked ham through the leek mixture.

9. Spoon the filling over the pastry base.

10. Beat the eggs with milk and a pinch of black pepper, grate in cheese.

11. Pour over the vegetables and ham.

12. Place grate over the rest of the cheese.

13. Place the baking tray, let bake for 30 minutes.

14. Let rest for 15 minutes, serve and enjoy.

Leek, potato, and pea soup

Ingredients

- A few sprigs of fresh flat-leaf parsley
- 2 large leeks
- 200g of frozen peas
- 1 large potato
- 1½ tablespoons of olive oil
- 1 teaspoon of bouillon powder
- 400ml of milk

Directions

1. Begin by heating olive oil over medium heat.
2. Then, add the leek together with the potatoes, fry for 5 minutes.
3. Add the bouillon powder.
4. Pour in 400ml water, reduce the heat, simmer for 10 minutes.
5. Add the milk together with the parsley and peas to the pan, simmer for a further 5 minutes to warm through.
6. Serve and enjoy.

Chickpea, leek, and carrot stew

Ingredients

- ½ tablespoon of olive oil
- 1 small leek
- 1 small carrot
- 2 tablespoons of natural yoghurt
- 1 x 210g tin of chickpeas

Directions

1. Heat olive oil in a medium pan over medium heat.
2. Add the leek, let cook until softened, then add the carrots with 200ml water.
3. Bring to the boil, when covered, then reduce to a simmer for until the vegetables are tender.
4. Drain, then add the chickpeas, let warm through for 5 minutes, then remove.
5. Let cool briefly, then stir through the yoghurt.
6. Mash until fairly smooth, with some soft lumps.
7. Serve and enjoy.

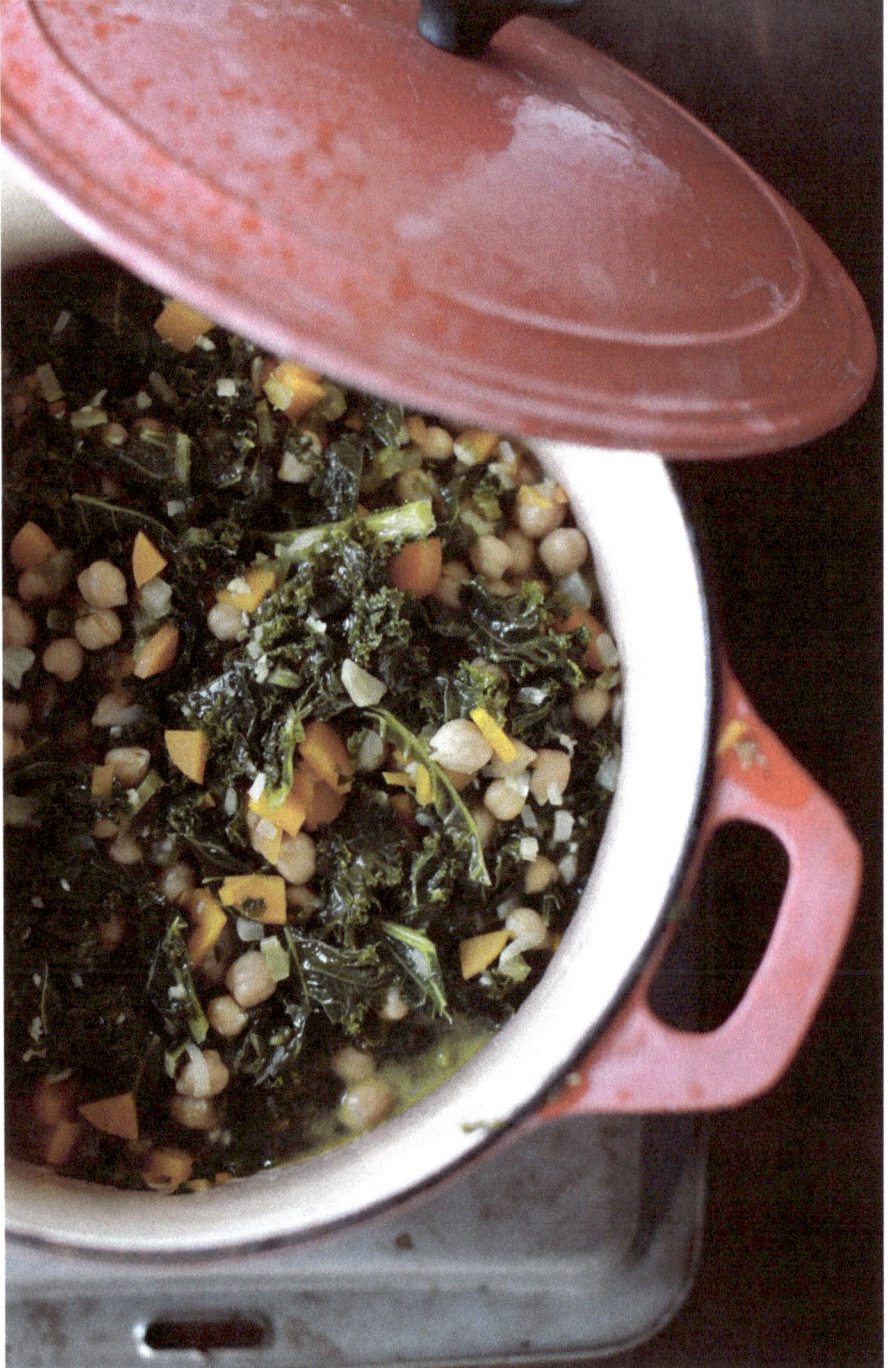

.

www.ingramcontent.com/pod-product-compliance
Lightning Source LLC
Chambersburg PA
CBHW062343300326
41947CB00012B/1193